Today was a big day. It was Sammy's first day at big school and he was filled with a lot of different feelings. He felt excited when he thought of all the friends he would make.

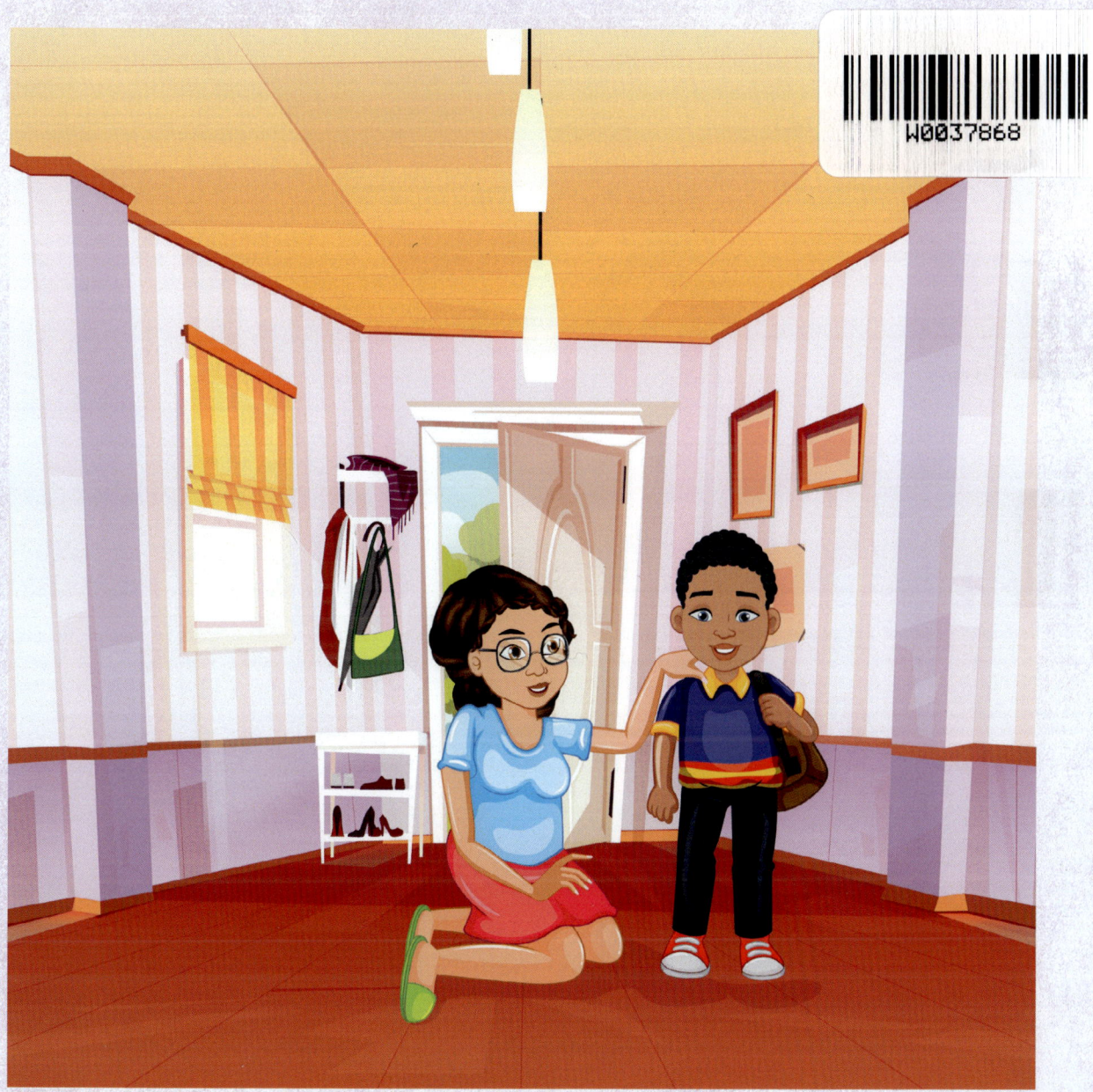

He felt really happy when he thought about everything he was going to learn. But . . . He also felt a little nervous, a little scared, and a little quiet.

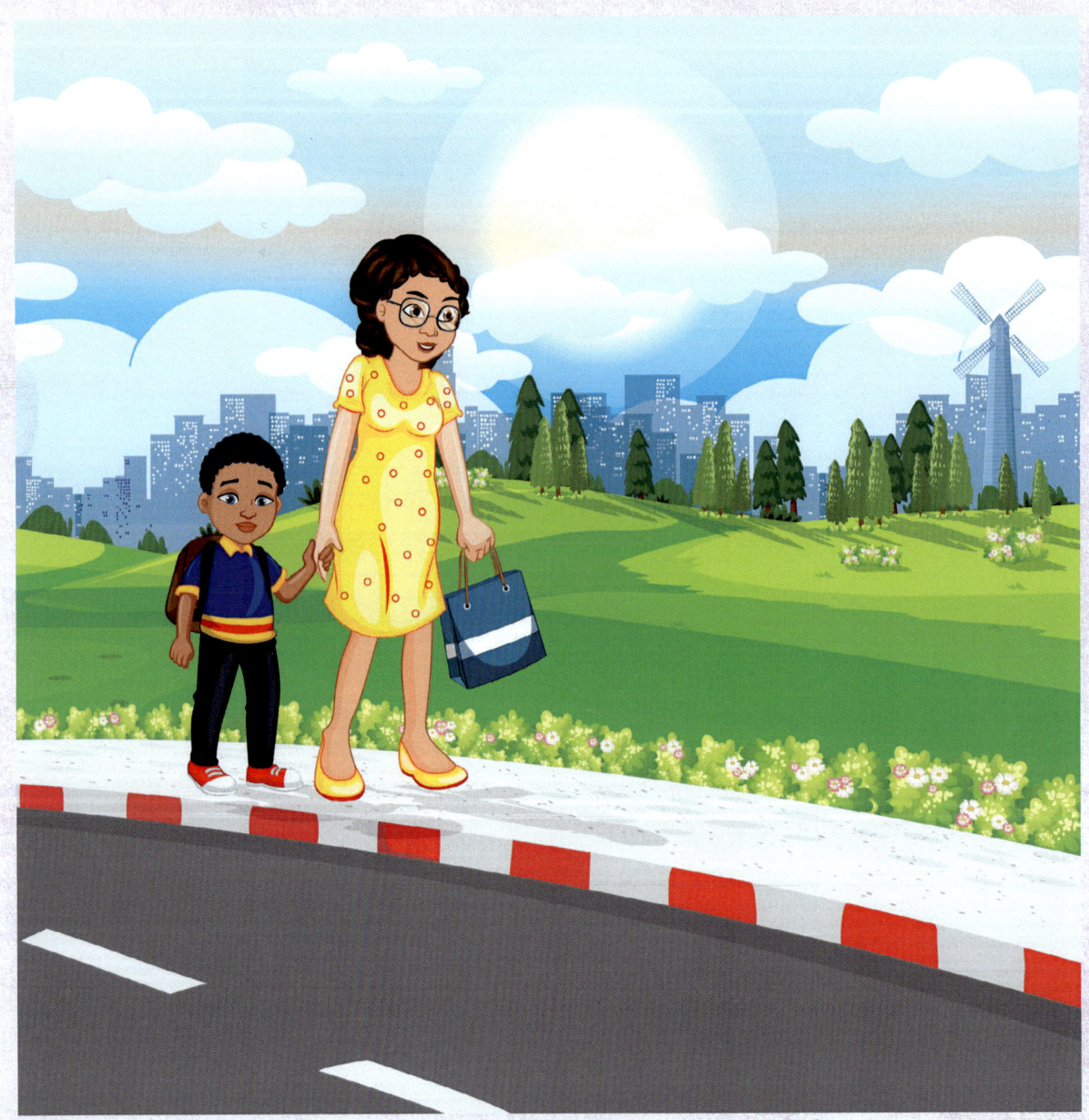

"That's OK," said Sammy's mom as they both walked to the school gates.
"It's normal to feel a little bit scared. Just remember the most important things:
be positive, be understanding, and be kind. You'll make lots of friends; I just know it!"

Sammy and his mom both took a big breath in and let a big breath out.
Now he felt nice and calm. Just as Sammy was about to go,
his mom grabbed his hand. "This is for you," she said, handing him a flower.

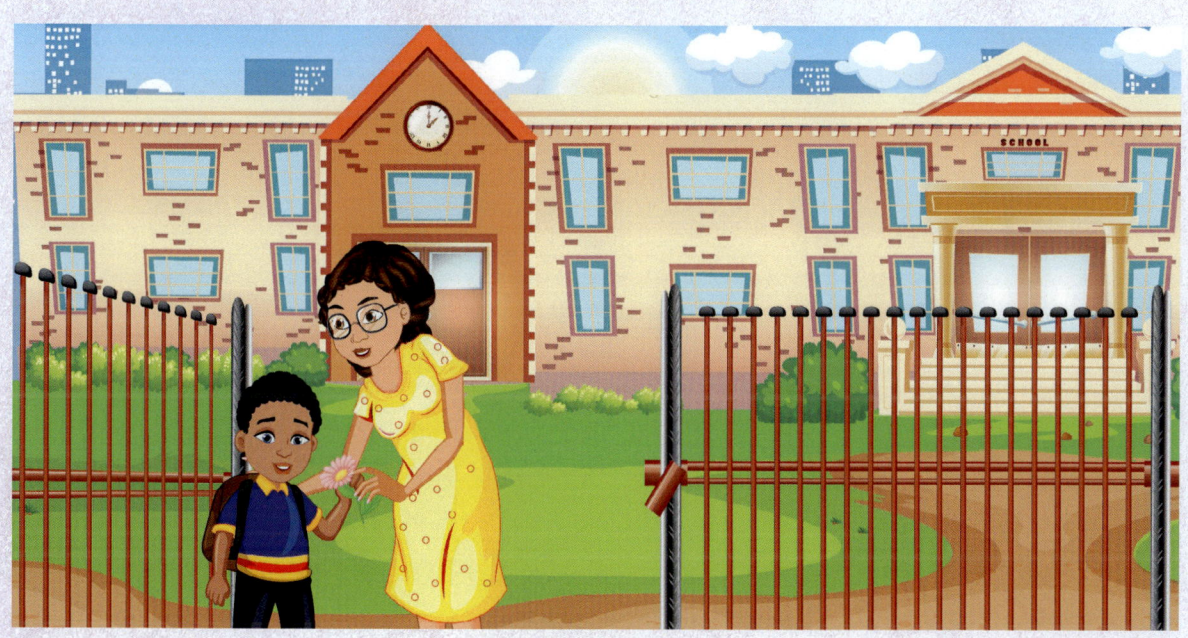

Sammy waved goodbye to his mom and skipped off into school.
He could already see so many other kids, all as excited and nervous as he was.
He couldn't wait to get inside and meet them all!

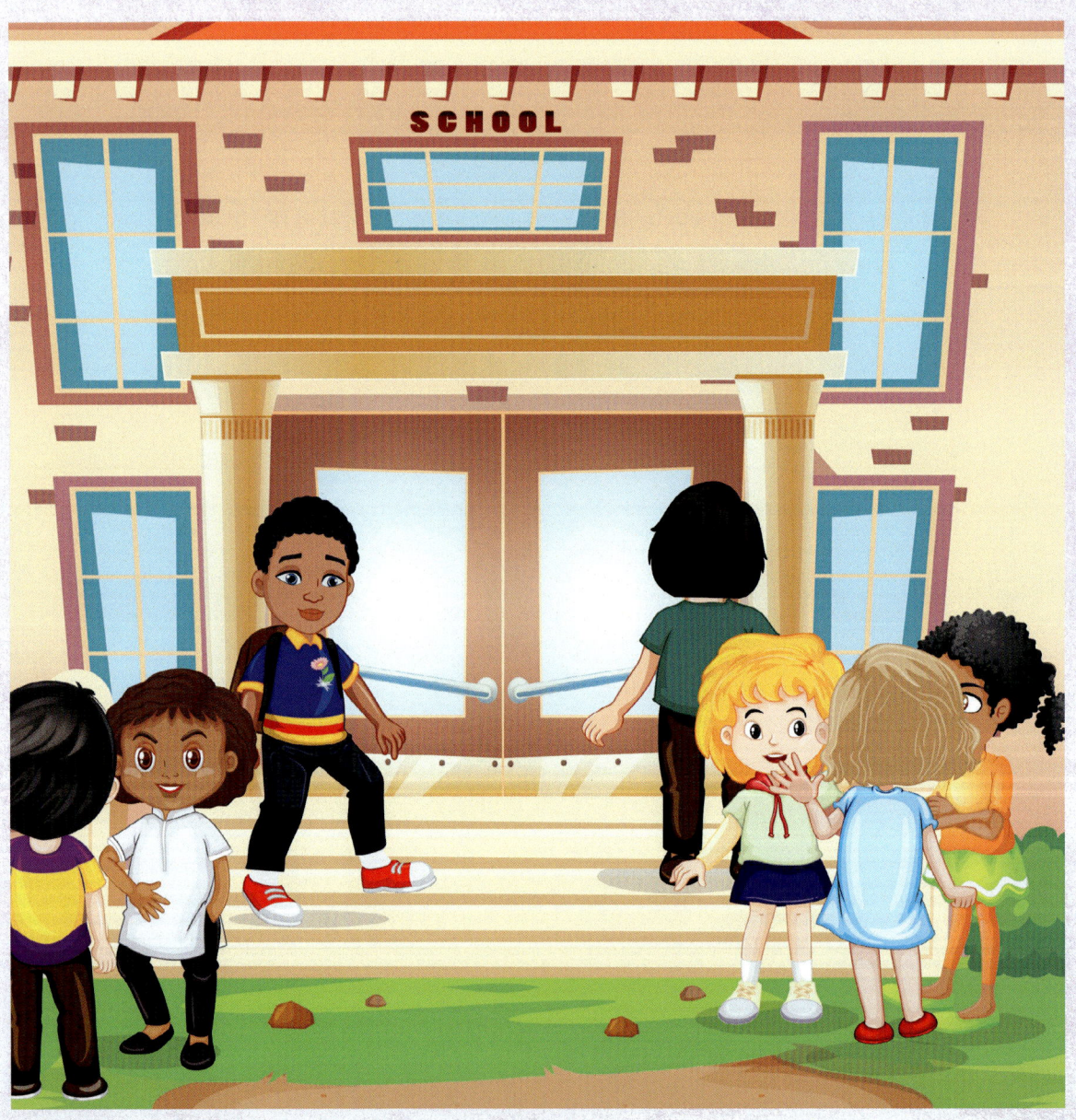

"Be positive, be understanding, and be kind," Sammy said to himself and took a big step through the entrance. It was a little bit scary, with so many people around. There was so much happening already.

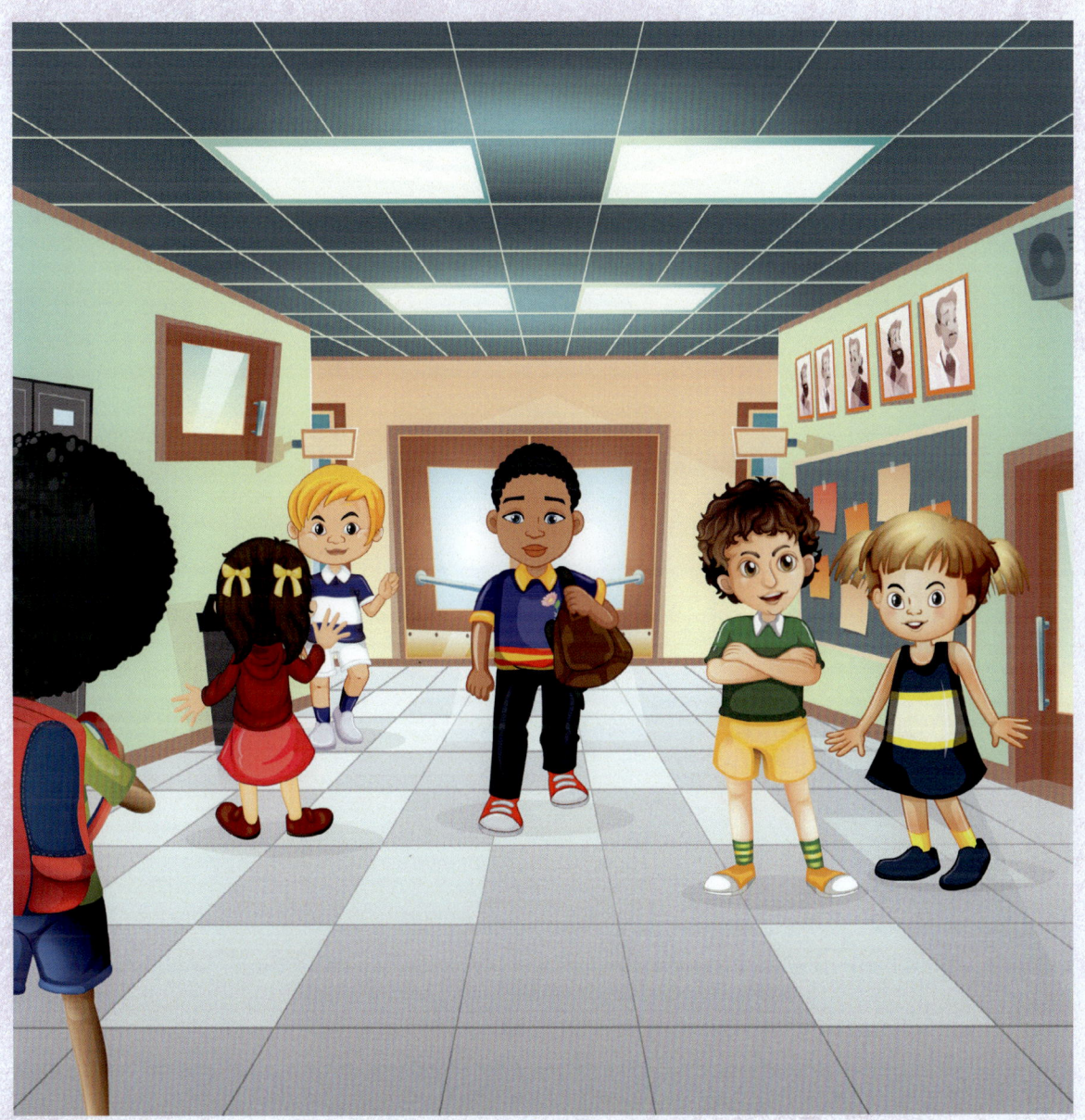

Lots of people were talking together. They were smiling and laughing
and making friends. Suddenly, Sammy started to feel a little nervous,
a little scared, and a little quiet. But then he saw something . . .

A girl was trying to hang up her coat, but she couldn't quite reach all the way to
the hook. In a flash, Sammy rushed over and asked her if she needed help.
"Thanks," said the girl, as Sammy hung it up for her. "My name's Lucy."

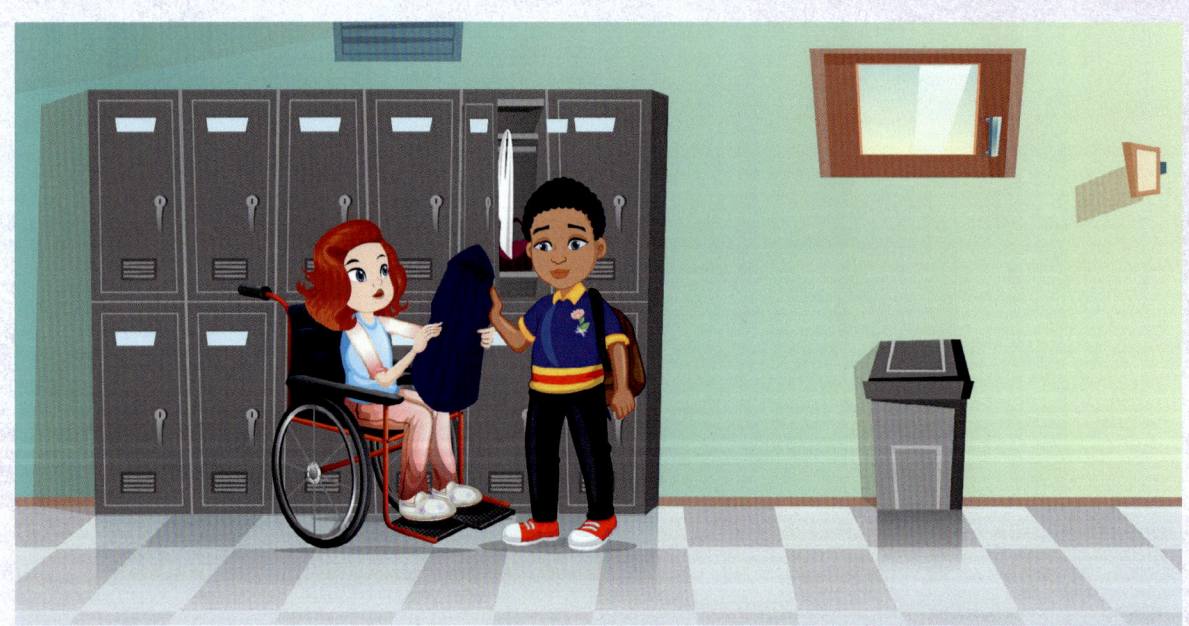

"I'm Sammy," he replied, and the two of them went into class and sat right next to each other. This is great! Sammy thought. I've already made a friend! Then another boy sat beside him, too. But when Sammy went to say hello . . .

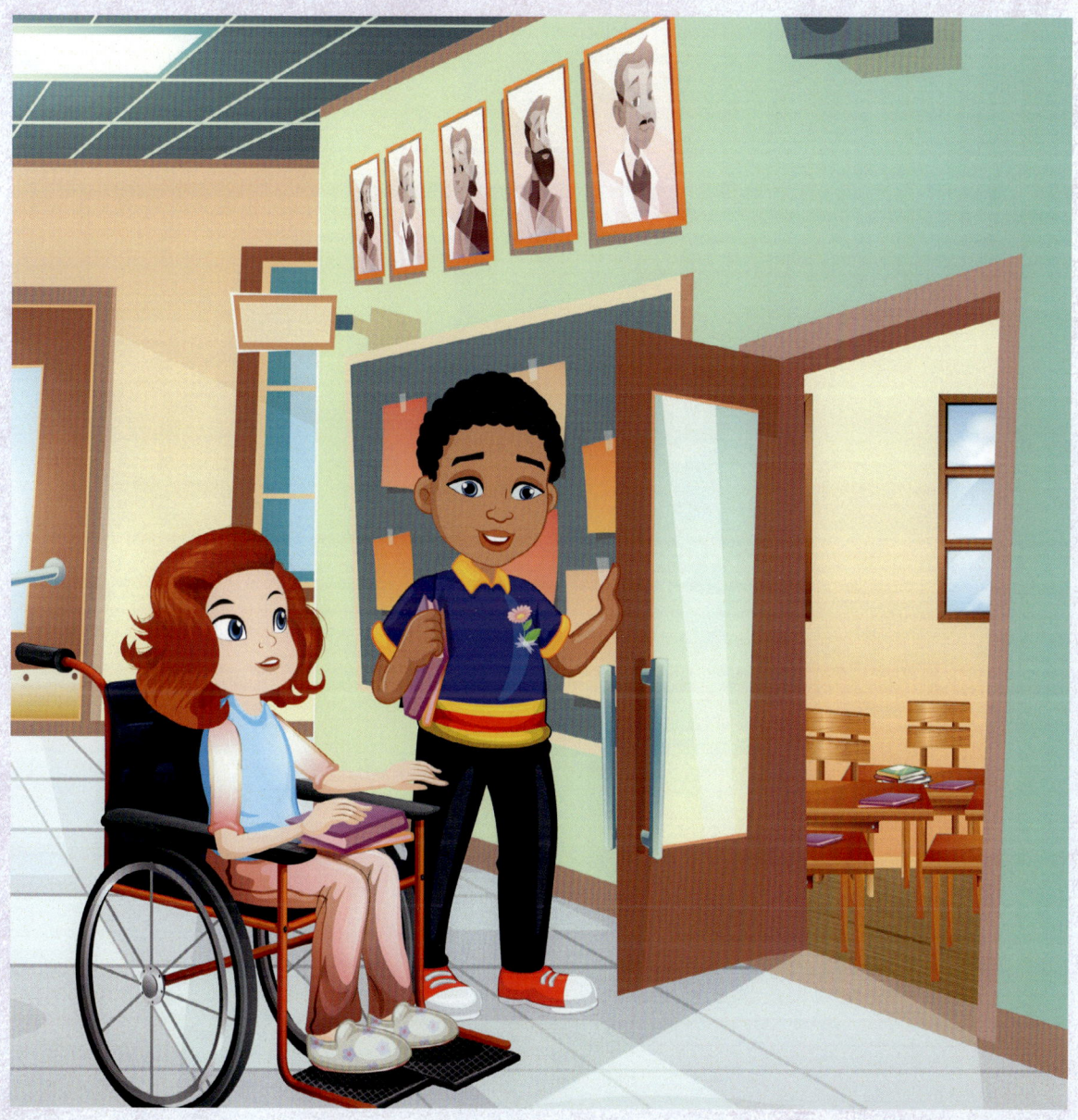

Sammy saw that the boy seemed very worried. He was looking under the desk, checking in his pockets, and searching through his bag. "Are you OK?" Sammy asked, taking the boy by surprise.

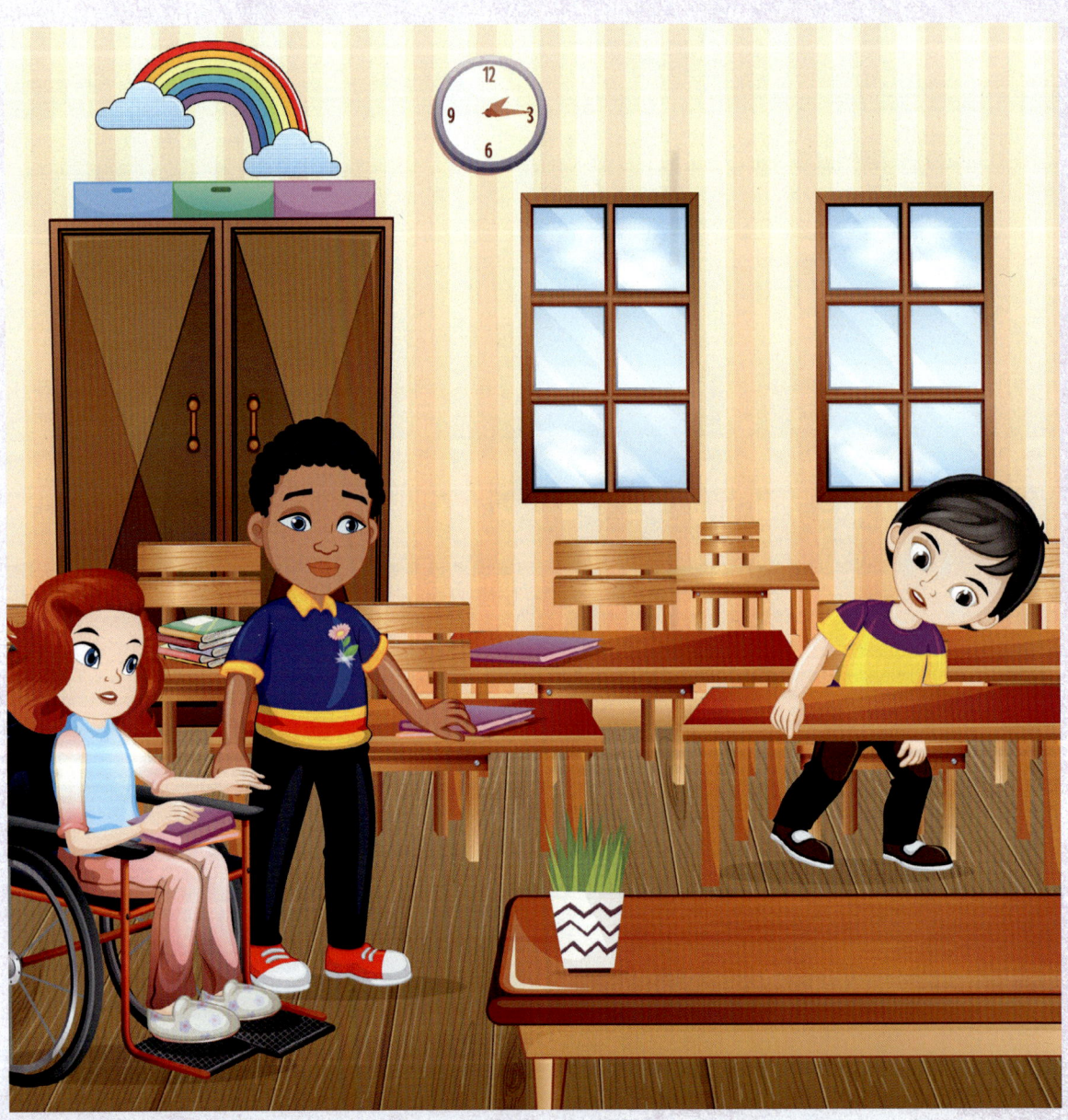

"I've lost my pencil," he said, looking very upset.

"I knew something would go wrong today and it already has."

But Sammy knew what to do. He took a deep breath in and let a deep breath out.

The boy did the same, and soon he was feeling calm again.

Reaching into his bag, Sammy took out a spare pencil and gave it to him.

"You can have mine!" he announced, smiling wide.

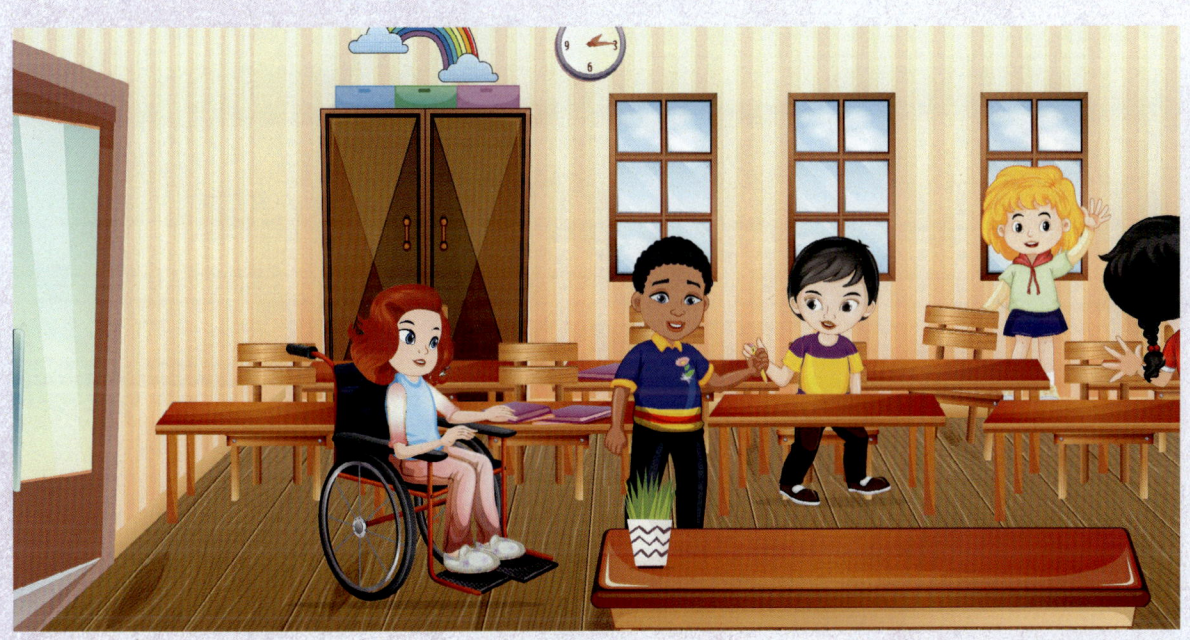

"Thanks!" said the boy. "My name is Mo." Sammy introduced Mo to Lucy and soon the three of them were laughing and joking together. Sammy was starting to forget why he had felt nervous at all.

As the morning went by, Sammy made more and more friends. Whenever anybody needed help, or a favor, or even a smile, Sammy was there to be their friend.

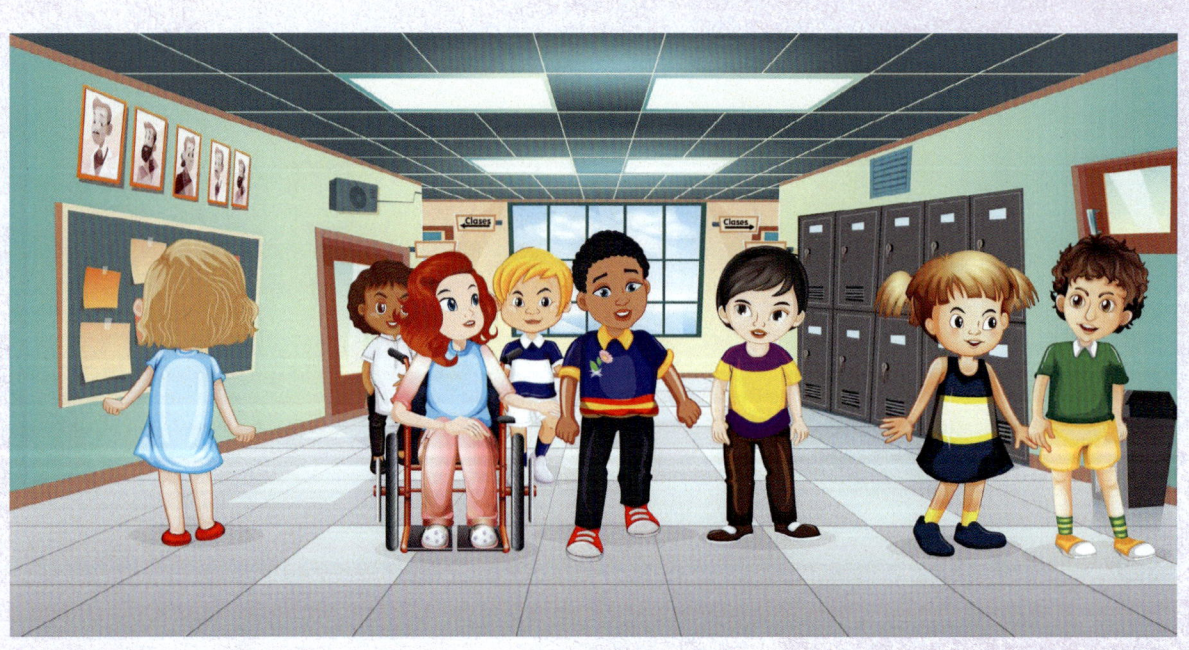

By the time lunchtime came, Sammy was sitting and eating with a whole group of new friends. They all said that they had started the day feeling very nervous, but now they felt much better. But as everyone was getting to know each other . . .

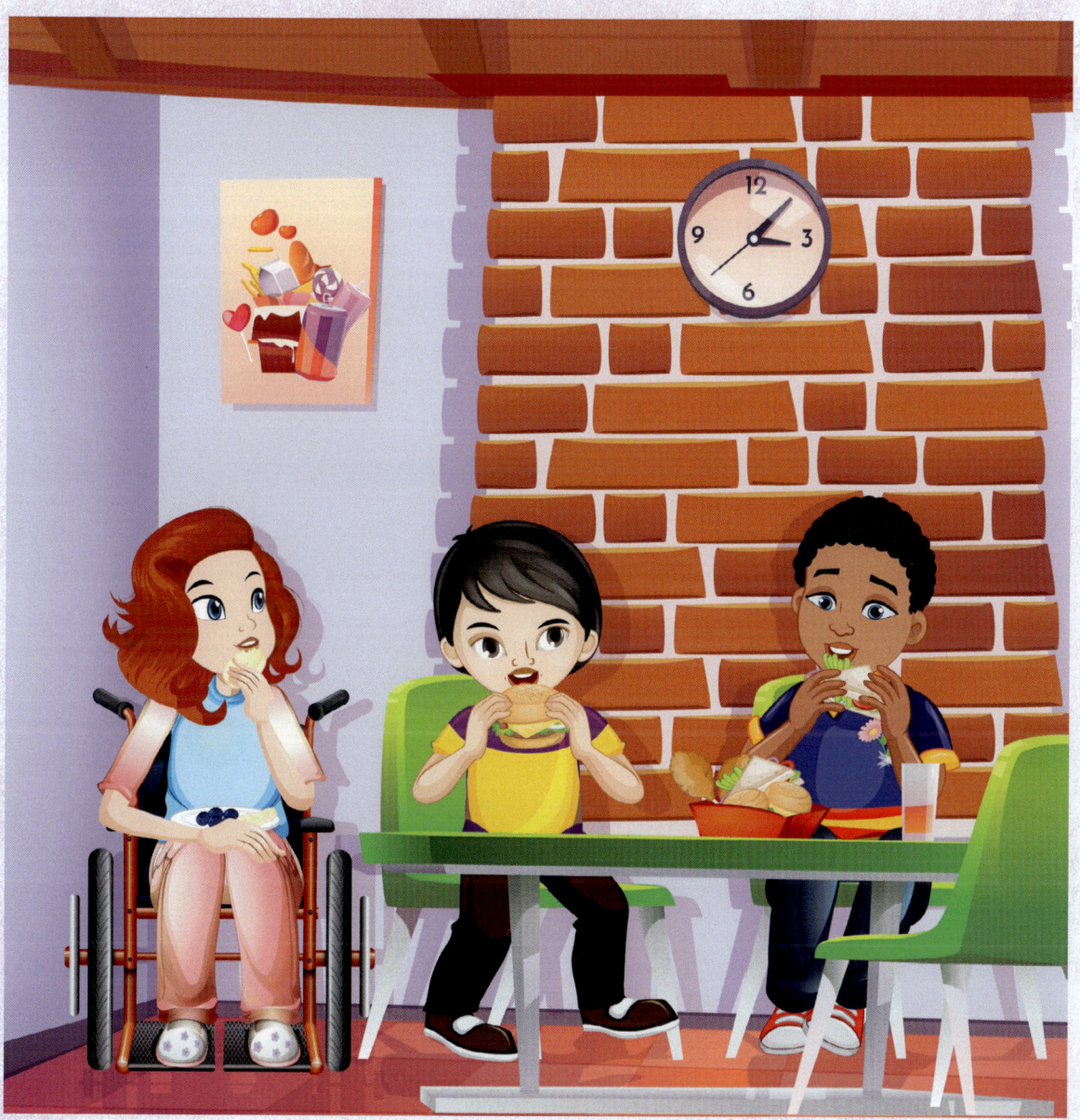

Sammy couldn't help but notice someone sitting all alone at another table.
It was a girl in his class, but no one had talked to her all day.
She'd been very quiet and hadn't made any friends yet.

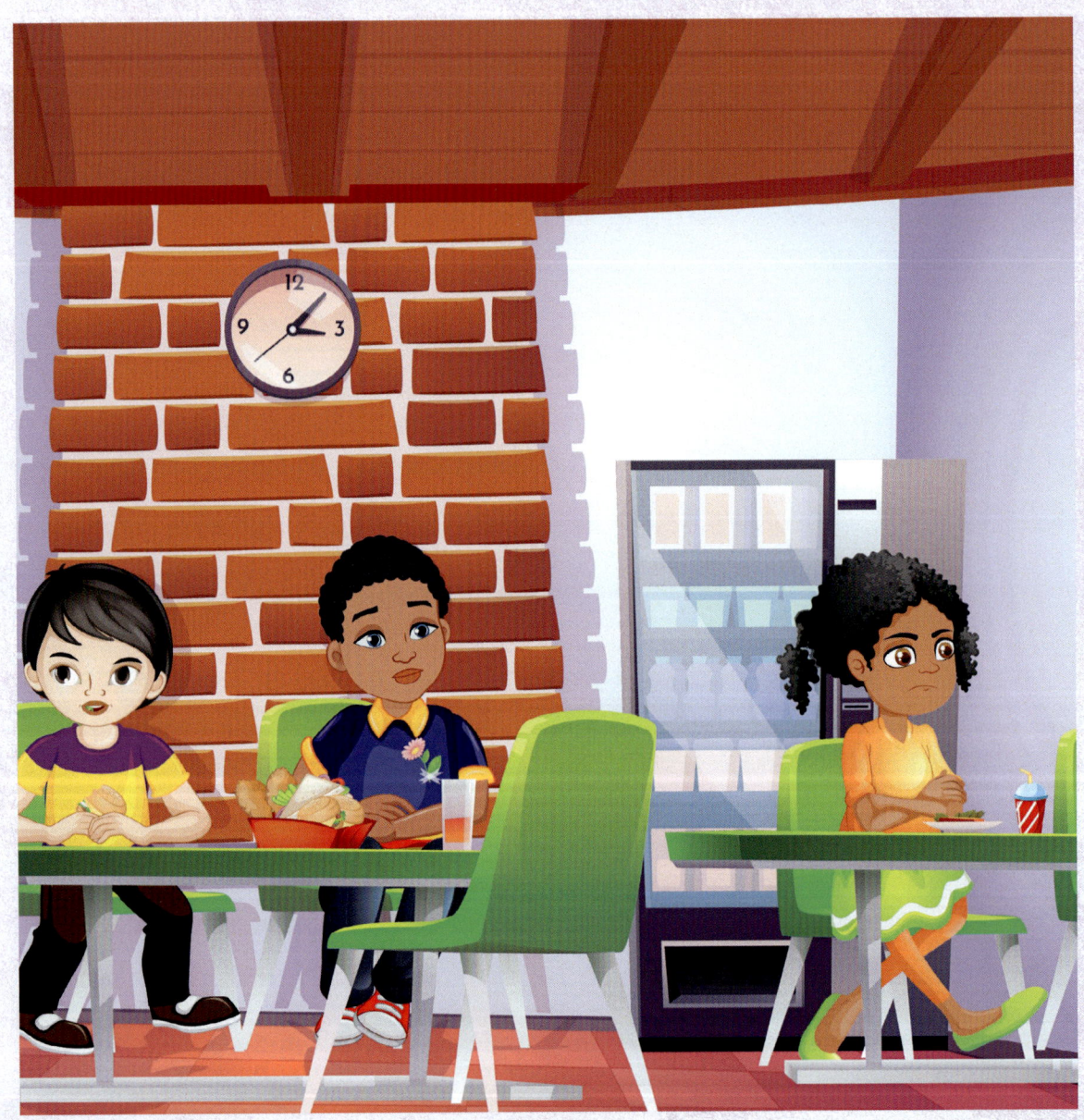

"She pushed in front of me in the line," someone complained. "She ignored me when I sat next to her," huffed someone else. "I don't think she's very nice," announced another kid. But the more Sammy looked at her, the more he started to think . . .

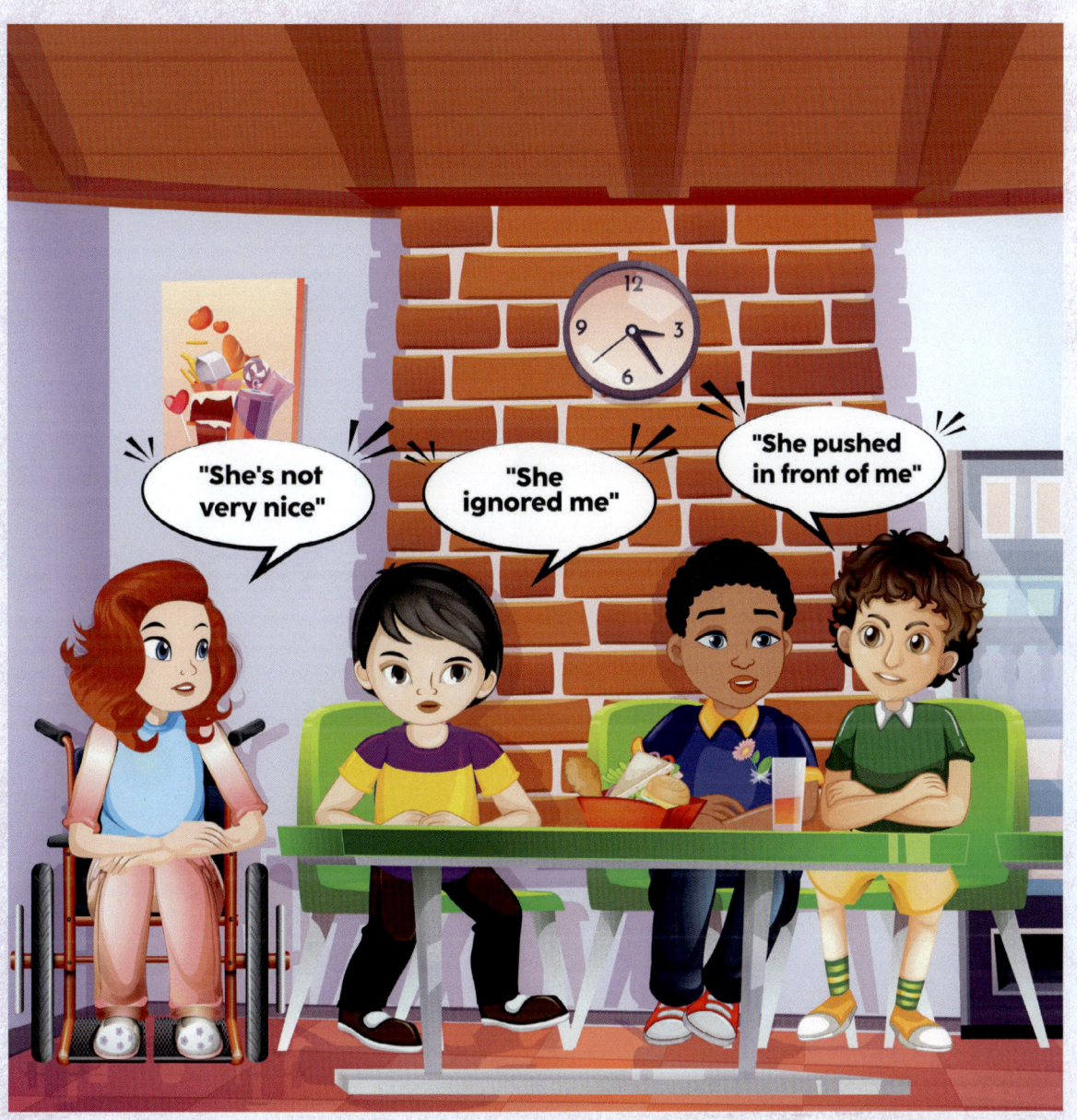

Sammy walked over and sat down next to the girl. "I'm Sammy," he said. "What's your name?" At first, the girl didn't say anything. She just ate her lunch in silence. Sammy wasn't sure what to do next.

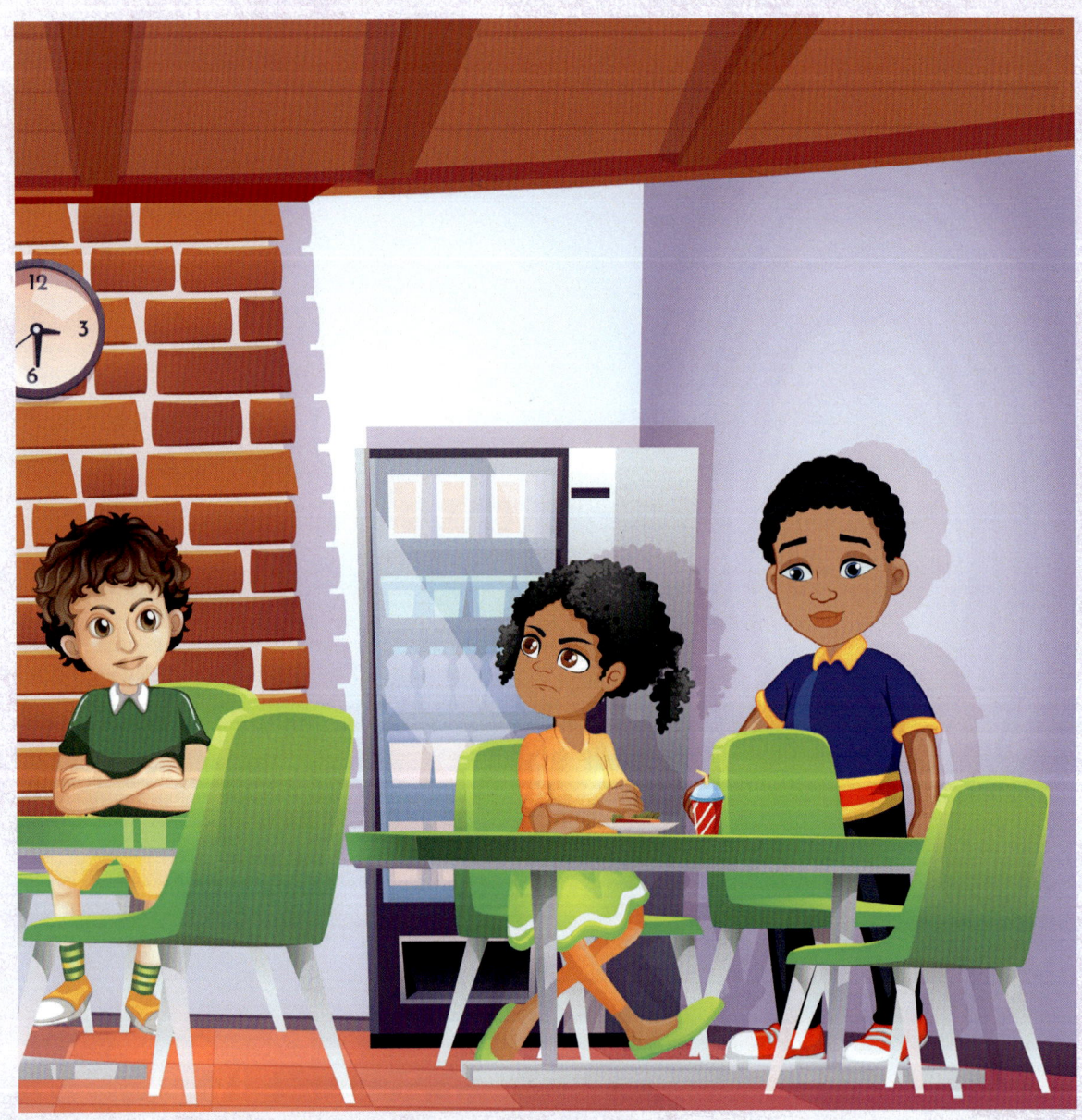

But then he remembered . . .

Be positive, be understanding, and be kind.
Taking the flower from his buttonhole, he held it up to the girl and smiled.

"It's OK," he said. "It's normal to feel a bit nervous, a bit scared, and a bit quiet.
This is for you." The girl took the flower and Sammy saw her smile.
She looked very relieved.

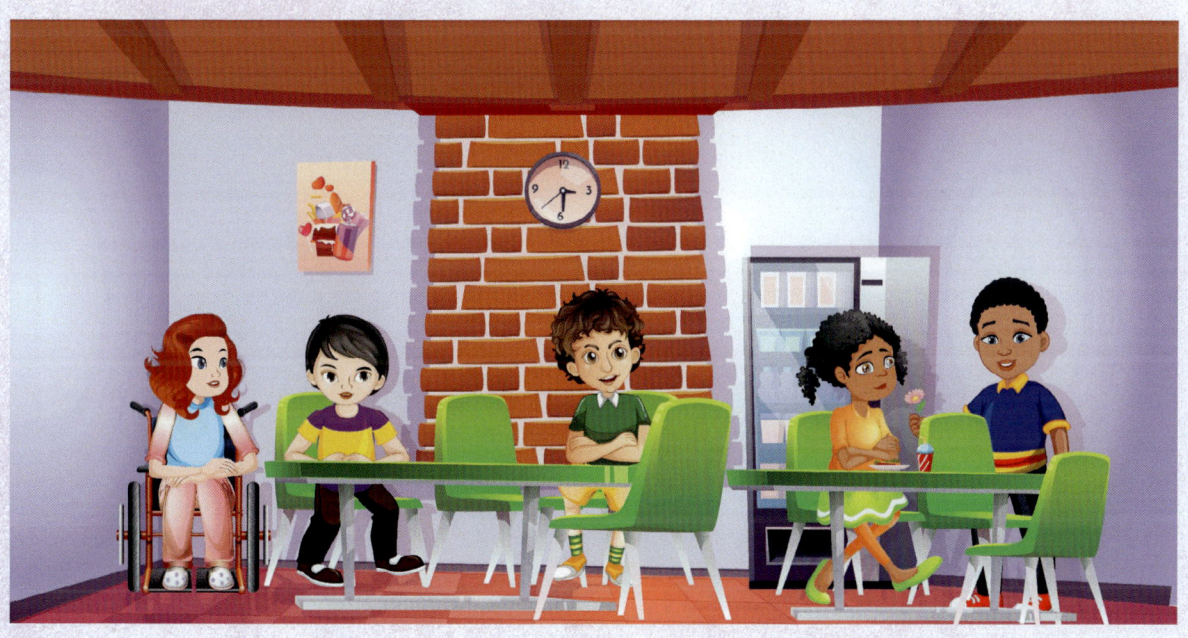

"I didn't mean to be unkind," she said. "I was just so worried that I wouldn't make any friends." "I felt the same," Sammy said, and then he had a great idea.

"Take a deep breath with me." They both took a deep breath in and a deep breath out.

"All you need to do is remember to be positive, be understanding, and be kind," said Sammy, and a smile spread across the girl's face. "Then people will be kind to you." "My name is Ava," she said.

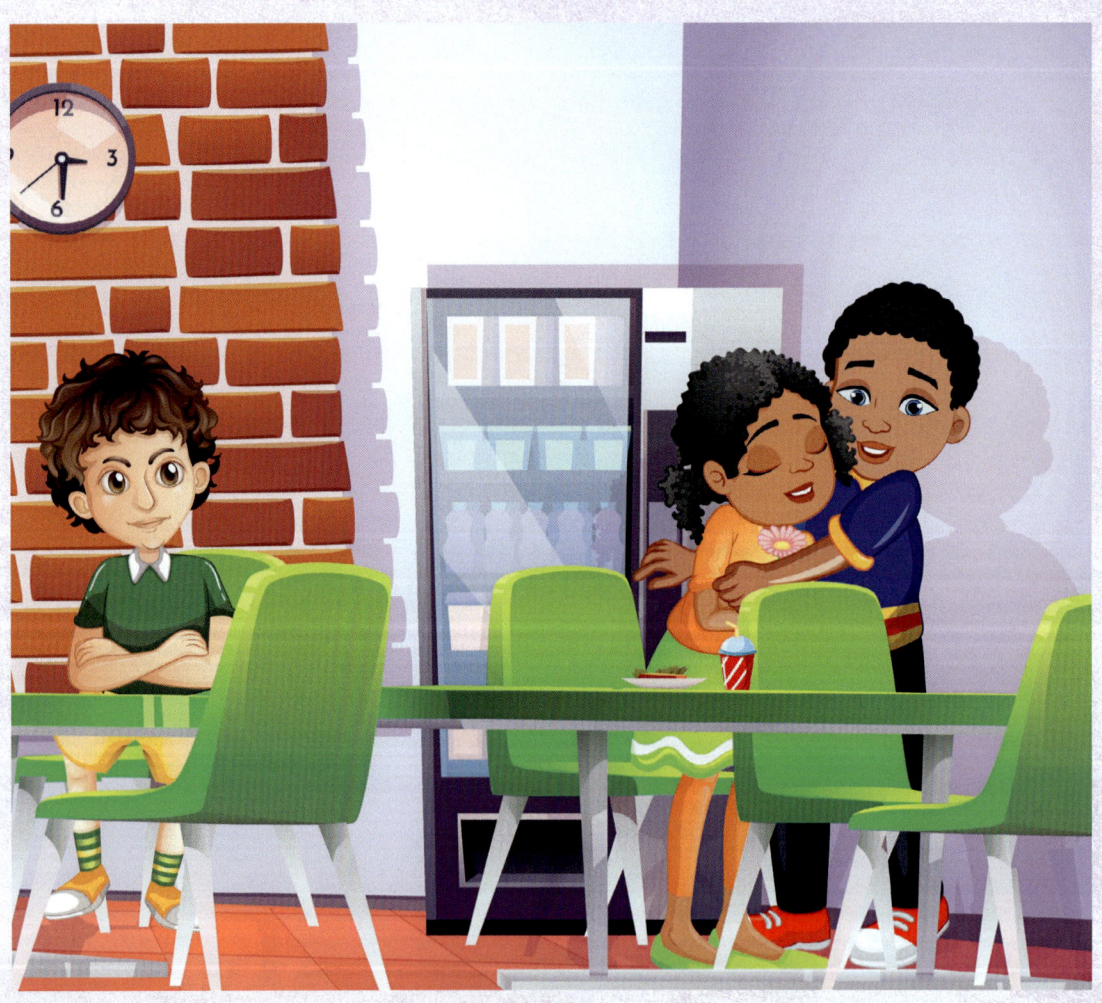

When Sammy introduced his new friend to everyone, they were all so happy to meet her. They had many things in common, and Ava's mom had even baked cookies for her to share with the whole class.

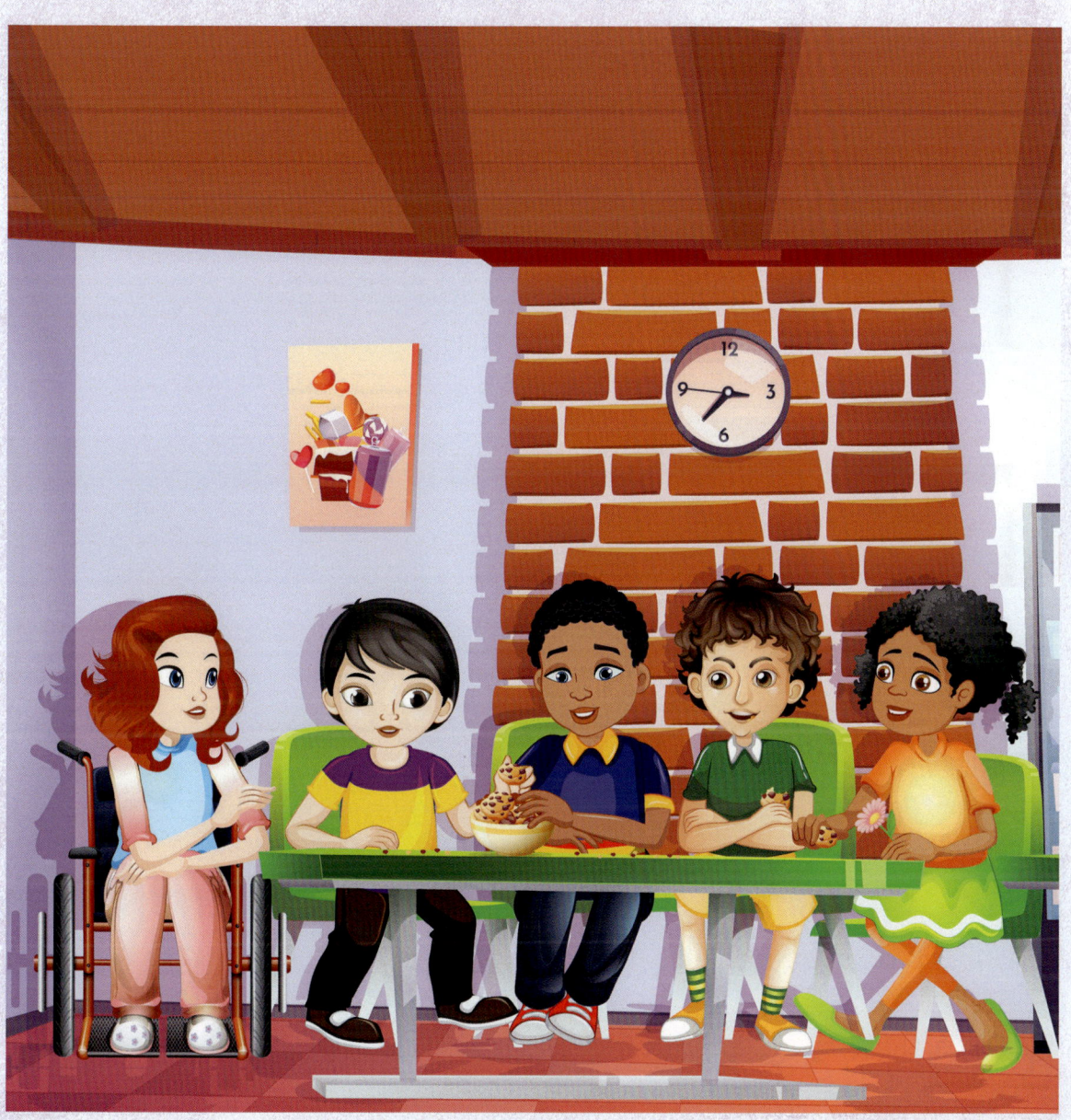

When the first day was over, Sammy waved goodbye to all of his new friends.

"See you tomorrow," said Lucy.

"See you later!" said Mo.

"Goodbye, Sammy!" called Ava, holding her flower up in the air.

"How was your day?" Sammy's mom asked as they made their way back home.

"I felt a bit nervous, a bit scared, and a bit quiet at first," Sammy admitted.

"But then I remembered what you told me and suddenly everything was fine."

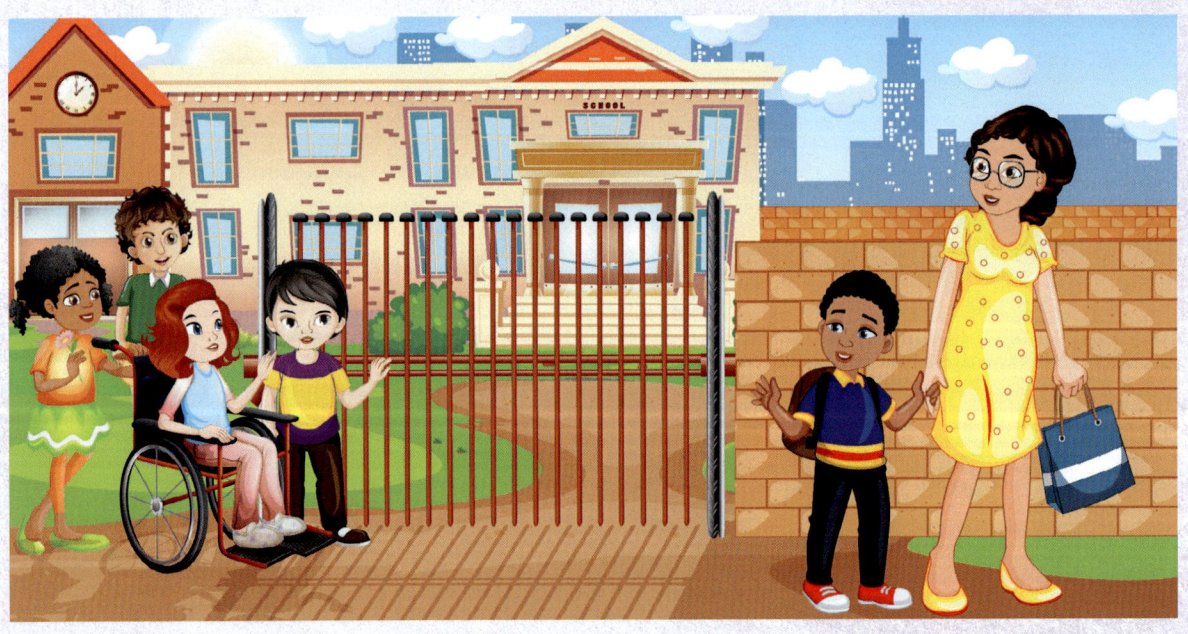

When Sammy got home, he was already looking forward to going back tomorrow.
But now there was one last person that he had to be kind to.

He plucked a fresh flower from the garden.

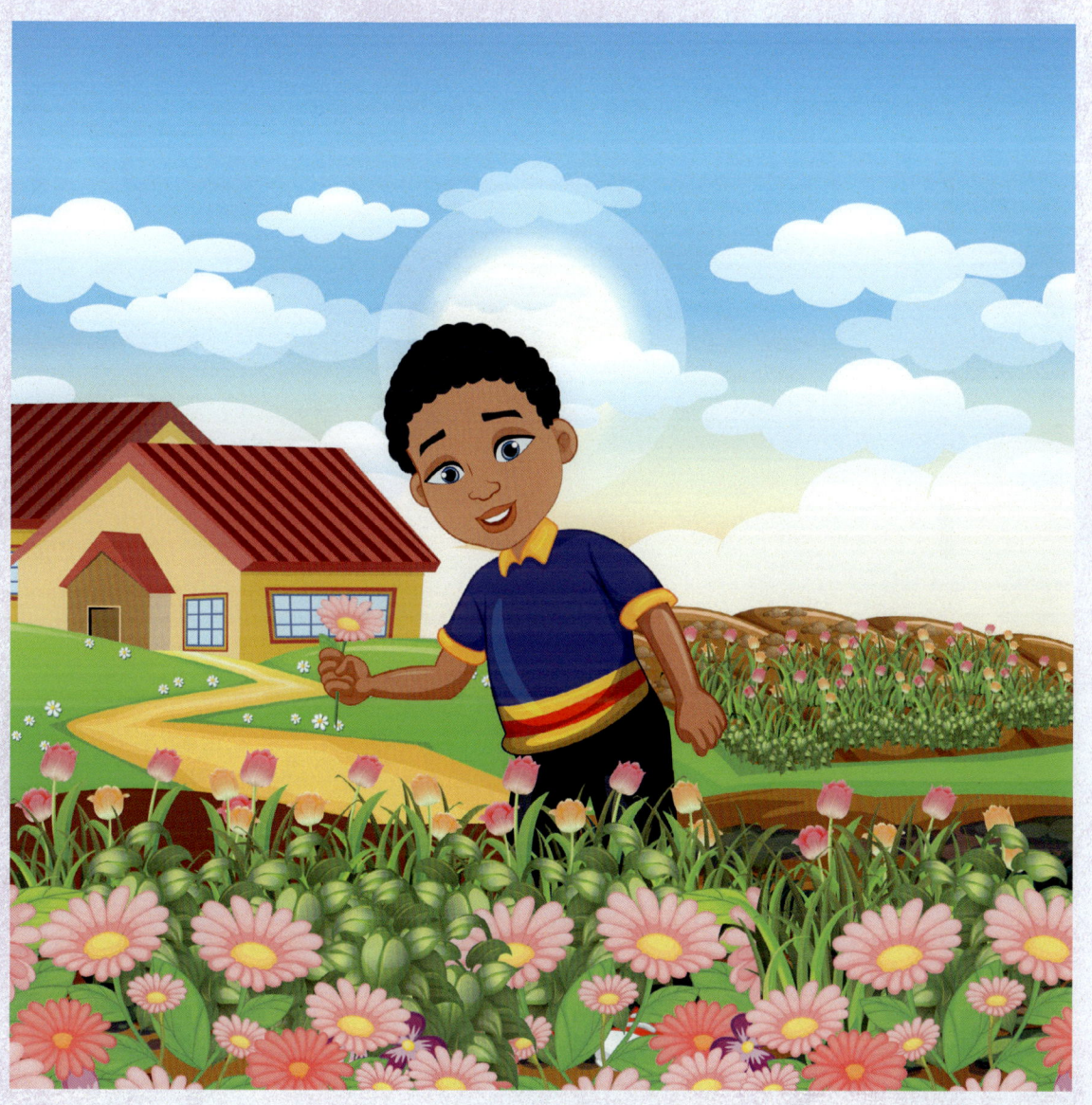

Then he laid back on the couch and read his favorite book.
Now was the time to be kind to himself. What a big day it had been!

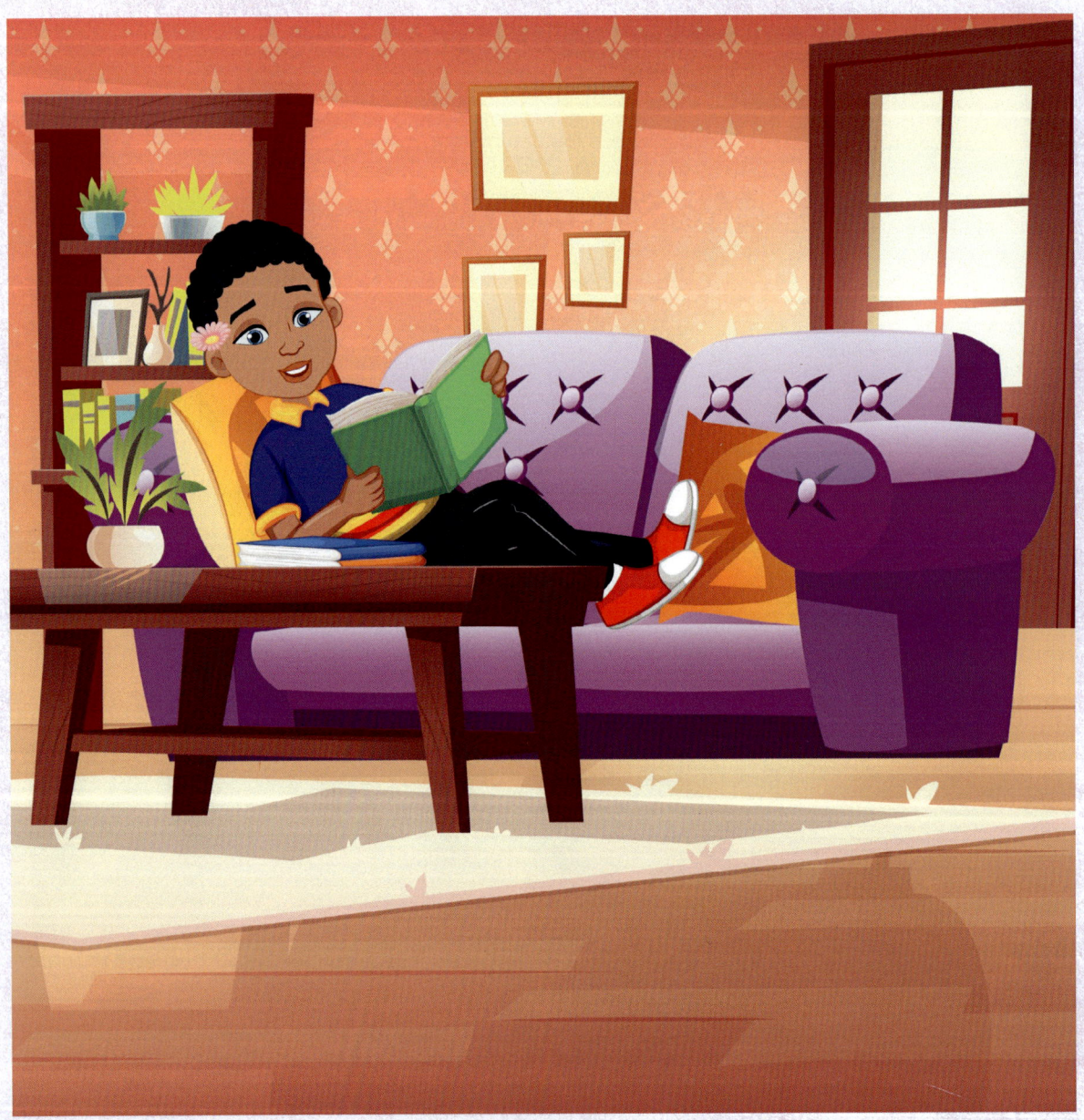